SURVIVING PROSTATE CANCER

A Survivor's Guide to Beating Prostate Cancer

Edward K. Jones

All rights reserved. No part of this publication may be reproduced, distributed, or transmitted in any form or by any means, including photocopying, recording, or other electronic or mechanical methods, without the prior written permission of the publisher, except in the case of brief quotations embodied in critical reviews and certain other noncommercial uses permitted by copyright law.

Copyright © Edward K. Jones, 2023.

Table Of Contents

Chapter 1
Introduction
Purpose of the Guide
My Personal Story

Chapter 2
Understanding Prostate Cancer: What is Prostate Cancer?
Causes and Risk Factors
Symptoms and Warning Signs
How is Prostate Cancer Diagnosed?
Stages of Prostate Cancer
Types of Prostate Cancer

Chapter 3
Treatment Options: Surgery
Radical Prostatectomy
Robotic-Assisted Laparoscopic Prostatectomy
Radiation Therapy
External Beam Radiation Therapy
Brachytherapy (Seed Implants)
Hormone Therapy
Androgen Deprivation Therapy (ADT)
Chemotherapy
Watchful Waiting or Active Surveillance
Clinical Trials

Chapter 4
Coping with Treatment Side Effects
Common Side Effects of Prostate Cancer Treatment: Urinary Incontinence
Erectile Dysfunction
Hot Flashes
Tips for Managing Side Effects
Alternative and Complementary Therapies

Chapter 5
Lifestyle Changes for a Healthy Recovery: Nutrition and Diet
Exercise and Physical Activity
Stress Management and Relaxation Techniques
Sleep and Rest
Smoking Cessation and Alcohol Moderation

Chapter 6
Emotional Support and Coping Strategies: Understanding the Emotional Impact of Prostate Cancer
Coping with Anxiety and Depression
Building a Support System
Support Groups and Counseling

Chapter 7
Follow-Up Care and Surveillance: Monitoring for Recurrence
Prostate-Specific Antigen (PSA) Testing
Imaging Tests

Understanding Test Results

Chapter 8
Advocacy and Education: Advocating for Yourself and Others
Prostate Cancer Research and Advocacy Organizations
Staying Up-to-Date on Prostate Cancer News and Research

Chapter 9
Resources for Prostate Cancer Survivors: Financial Assistance and Insurance
Legal and Employment Issues
Transportation and Lodging

Chapter 10
Inspiring Survivor Stories

Conclusion

Chapter 1

Introduction

Prostate cancer is a type of cancer that develops in the prostate gland, a small walnut-structured gland located below the bladder in men. The prostate gland is part of the male reproductive system and produces fluid that forms a part of semen. Prostate cancer occurs when the cells in the prostate gland grow and divide uncontrollably, forming a tumor.

Prostate cancer is the most common cancer in men, other than skin cancer, and it is estimated that 1 in every 8 men will be diagnosed with prostate cancer during their lifetime. The majority of prostate cancers are slow-growing and may not cause any symptoms or problems. However, some types of prostate cancer can be aggressive and spread to other parts of the body, which can be life-threatening.

The causes of prostate cancer are not well understood, but several risk factors increase the likelihood of developing prostate cancer. Age is the most significant risk factor, with the risk of developing prostate cancer increasing with age. Other risk factors include family history, race, and certain genetic mutations.

Prostate cancer can cause a variety of symptoms, although in many cases, there are no symptoms at all. Symptoms of prostate cancer may include difficulty urinating, weak or interrupted urine flow, blood in the urine or semen, pain or discomfort in the pelvic area, and erectile dysfunction.

Prostate cancer is typically diagnosed through a combination of a physical exam, a blood test to measure prostate-specific antigen (PSA) levels, and a biopsy of the prostate gland. Once prostate cancer has been diagnosed, the stage of the cancer is determined to guide treatment decisions. The stages of prostate cancer range from Stage I, where the cancer is confined to the prostate gland, to Stage IV, where the cancer has spread to other parts of the body.

There are several treatment options for prostate cancer, including surgery, radiation remedy, hormone remedy, and chemotherapy. The choice of treatment depends on the stage and type of prostate cancer, as well as the overall health of the patient. With early detection and appropriate treatment, many men with prostate cancer can live long, healthy lives.

Purpose of the Guide

Prostate cancer is one of the most common cancers in men worldwide. It's estimated that 1 in every 8 men will be diagnosed with prostate cancer during their continuance. Prostate cancer can be a scary diagnosis, but it is important to remember that it is treatable and even curable in many cases.

As a survivor of prostate cancer, I understand the physical, emotional, and mental toll that a prostate cancer diagnosis can take on a person and their loved ones. I decided to write this guide to share my experience and provide helpful information and resources for other men who are battling prostate cancer.

The purpose of this guide is to serve as a comprehensive resource for men who have been diagnosed with prostate cancer, their families, and their caregivers. This guide covers all aspects of prostate cancer, including understanding the disease, treatment options, coping with side effects, making lifestyle changes, emotional support, follow-up care, advocacy and education, resources for survivors, and inspiring survivor stories.

In the first section of this guide, we will provide an overview of prostate cancer. We will discuss what prostate cancer is, the causes and risk factors associated with it, and the common symptoms and warning signs to watch out for. We will also cover how prostate cancer is diagnosed and the different stages and types of prostate cancer that exist.

In the second section, we will dive into the various treatment options available for prostate cancer. We will cover surgical options, such as radical prostatectomy and robotic-assisted laparoscopic prostatectomy, as well as radiation therapy and hormone therapy. We will also discuss watchful waiting or active surveillance and clinical trials for prostate cancer treatment.

The third section of this guide will focus on coping with treatment side effects. We will cover common side effects of prostate cancer treatment, including urinary incontinence, erectile dysfunction, fatigue, hot flashes, and nausea and vomiting. We will provide tips for managing these side effects and discuss alternative and complementary therapies that may be helpful.

The fourth section will discuss lifestyle changes that men can make to promote a healthy recovery from prostate cancer. We will cover nutrition and diet, exercise and physical activity, stress management and relaxation techniques, sleep and rest, and smoking cessation and alcohol moderation.

The fifth section of this guide will provide information on emotional support and coping strategies for men and their loved ones. We will discuss the emotional impact of prostate cancer and provide tips for coping with anxiety and depression. We will also cover building a support system, support groups, and counseling.

In the sixth section, we will cover follow-up care and surveillance for prostate cancer. We will discuss monitoring for recurrence, PSA testing, imaging tests, understanding test results, and managing recurrence.

In the seventh section of this guide, we will discuss advocacy and education for prostate cancer survivors. We will provide tips for advocating for oneself and others, highlight prostate cancer research and advocacy organizations, and discuss ways to stay up-to-date on prostate cancer news and research.

The eighth section of this guide will provide resources for prostate cancer survivors, including financial assistance and insurance, legal and employment issues, transportation and lodging, clinical trials, and other support resources.

Finally, in the last section of this guide, we will share inspiring survivor stories. We will conduct interviews with prostate cancer survivors and share stories of hope and inspiration to help men and their loved ones navigate their prostate cancer journey.

I hope that this guide will be a valuable resource for men who have been diagnosed with prostate cancer and their families and caregivers. Remember, prostate cancer is treatable and even curable in many cases. With the right information, support, and resources, men can beat prostate cancer and live a fulfilling life after treatment.

My Personal Story

As a survivor of prostate cancer, I know firsthand the physical and emotional toll that this disease can take on a person and their loved ones. My journey with prostate cancer began when I noticed a gradual increase in difficulty with urination. At first, I dismissed it as a normal part of aging, but as the symptoms persisted and worsened, I knew that something was wrong.

I visited my primary care physician, who referred me to a urologist for further testing. The urologist performed a digital rectal exam and a blood test to measure my PSA levels. The results showed that my PSA levels were elevated, and a subsequent biopsy of my prostate gland confirmed the diagnosis of prostate cancer.

The news was overwhelming, and I felt a range of emotions, including fear, anger, and confusion. I was fortunate to have the support of my family and friends, who helped me navigate the treatment options and made sure that I received the best care possible.

After consulting with my urologist and an oncologist, we decided that surgery was the best course of action for me. I underwent a radical prostatectomy, which involved the complete removal of my prostate gland and surrounding tissue. The surgery was successful, and I was able to go home from the hospital after a few days.

The recovery process was challenging, both physically and emotionally. I experienced pain and discomfort, as well as urinary incontinence and erectile dysfunction. However, with the help of physical therapy and support from my healthcare team, I was able to regain my strength and adjust to the changes in my body.

In the years since my diagnosis and treatment, I have been vigilant about monitoring my PSA levels and visiting my healthcare provider regularly. I have also made lifestyle changes, such as eating a healthier diet and exercising regularly, to reduce my risk of recurrence.

My experience with prostate cancer has taught me the importance of early detection and treatment, as well as the value of a strong support system. I am grateful for the care that I received from my healthcare team and for the love and support of my family and friends. Through sharing my story, I hope to raise awareness about prostate cancer and encourage other men to take charge of their health and seek medical attention if they notice any unusual symptoms.

Chapter 2

Understanding Prostate Cancer: What is Prostate Cancer?

Prostate cancer is a type of cancer that occurs in the prostate gland, which is a small gland located below the bladder in men. The prostate gland is part of the male reproductive system and produces fluid that helps to nourish and transport sperm during ejaculation.

Prostate cancer develops when the cells in the prostate gland start to grow and divide abnormally, forming a tumor. In some cases, the cancer cells can spread to other parts of the body, such as the lymph nodes, bones, or other organs, which can be life-threatening.

The exact cause of prostate cancer is not known, but several risk factors can increase a man's likelihood of developing the disease. Age is a major risk factor, with prostate cancer being most common in men over the age of 65. Family history of prostate cancer, African-American ethnicity, and certain genetic mutations can also increase the risk of developing prostate cancer.

Prostate cancer can cause a range of symptoms, although in some cases, there may be no symptoms at all. Symptoms of prostate cancer can include difficulty urinating, weak or interrupted urine flow, frequent urination (especially at night), blood in the urine or semen, pain or discomfort in the pelvic area, and erectile dysfunction.

Diagnosis of prostate cancer typically involves a combination of a physical exam, blood tests, and imaging tests, such as a transrectal ultrasound or a magnetic resonance imaging (MRI) scan. A biopsy of the prostate gland may also be necessary to confirm the diagnosis of prostate cancer.

Treatment options for prostate cancer depend on the stage and type of cancer, as well as the overall health of the patient. Treatment options may include surgery, radiation therapy, hormone therapy, or chemotherapy. A combination of treatments may be used in some cases

Prostate cancer is a serious disease, but with early detection and appropriate treatment, many men can live long and healthy lives. Regular check-ups with a healthcare provider and awareness of the risk factors and symptoms of prostate cancer can help with early detection and improved outcomes.

Causes and Risk Factors

The exact cause of prostate cancer is not fully understood, but researchers have identified several factors that can increase a man's risk of developing the disease. Understanding these risk factors can help men take steps to reduce their risk and detect prostate cancer early when it is most treatable.

Age is the most significant threat factor for prostate cancer. The disease is rare in men under the age of 40 but becomes more common as men get older. About 60% of cases are diagnosed in men over the age of 65. The reason for this is unclear, but it may be related to changes in hormone levels as men age.

A family history of prostate cancer is another significant risk factor. Men with a father, brother, or son who has been diagnosed with prostate cancer are at higher risk themselves. This risk increases if the family member was diagnosed at a young age or if multiple family members have been affected.

Race is also a factor in prostate cancer risk. African American men have the highest risk of developing prostate cancer, followed by Hispanic men. Asian American and Pacific Islander men have the lowest risk. The reasons for these differences are not fully understood but may be related to genetic and environmental factors.

Certain genetic mutations have been linked to an increased risk of prostate cancer. These mutations are rare, but men who carry them have a much higher risk of developing the disease. Testing for these mutations is not routinely done but may be recommended for men with a strong family history of prostate cancer.

Other risk factors for prostate cancer include obesity, smoking, and exposure to certain chemicals. There is some evidence to suggest that a diet high in fat and low in fruits and vegetables may increase the risk of prostate cancer, but more research is needed to confirm this.

It is important to note that having one or more of these risk factors does not mean that a man will develop prostate cancer. Many men with no known risk factors are diagnosed with the disease, and many men with several risk factors never develop prostate cancer.

Regular screening is the most effective way to detect prostate cancer early before it has spread to other parts of the body. Screening may involve a blood test to measure prostate-specific antigen (PSA) levels and a digital rectal exam to check for abnormalities in the prostate gland. The American Cancer Society recommends that men discuss the pros and cons of screening with their healthcare provider starting at age 50, or earlier if they have a family history of prostate cancer or other threat factors.

In addition to regular screening, there are steps that men can take to reduce their risk of developing prostate cancer. Maintaining a healthy weight, quitting smoking, and limiting exposure to chemicals and toxins can all help to reduce the risk. Eating a healthy diet that is high in fruits and vegetables and low in fat may also be beneficial.

In summary, prostate cancer is a complex disease with multiple risk factors. Age, family history, race, and genetics are among the most significant risk factors, but lifestyle factors such as diet and exposure to toxins may also play a role. Regular screening and adopting a healthy lifestyle can help men reduce their risk of developing prostate cancer and detect the disease early when it is most treatable.

Symptoms and Warning Signs

Prostate cancer is a type of cancer that affects men. It is often asymptomatic, meaning that it does not cause any noticeable symptoms in its early stages. However, as the cancer progresses, it may cause symptoms that can be uncomfortable or even painful. Men need to be aware of the symptoms and warning signs of prostate cancer so that they can seek medical attention if necessary.

The symptoms of prostate cancer can vary depending on the stage of the complaint. In its early stages, prostate cancer may not cause any symptoms at all. As the cancer grows, it may beget the following symptoms.

1. Difficulty urinating: Prostate cancer can cause the prostate gland to enlarge, which can put pressure on the urethra and make it difficult to urinate. Men with prostate cancer may experience weak or interrupted urine flow, a need to urinate frequently (especially at night), or a feeling of not being able to empty the bladder.

2. Blood in the urine or semen: Prostate cancer can cause blood vessels to break, which can result in blood in the urine or semen. This symptom is not always present, but if it does occur, it is important to seek medical attention.

3. Erectile dysfunction: Prostate cancer can affect the nerves and blood vessels that control the penis, which can lead to difficulty achieving or maintaining an erection.

4. Pain or discomfort: Prostate cancer can cause pain or discomfort in the prostate gland, the pelvic region, or other parts of the body. This symptom is more common in advanced cases of

prostate cancer, but it can occur at any stage of the disease.

It's important to note that these symptoms can also be caused by other conditions, similar to an enlarged prostate or a urinary tract infection. However, if any of these symptoms persist or worsen over time, it is important to see a healthcare provider for further evaluation.

In addition to the symptoms listed above, there are also some warning signs of prostate cancer that men should be aware of. These include:

1. Family history: Men with a family history of prostate cancer are at higher risk of developing the disease themselves.

2. Age: Prostate cancer is more common in men over the age of 50.

3. Race: African American men and men of Caribbean descent are at higher risk of

developing prostate cancer than men of other races.

4. Obesity: Men who are overweight or obese may be at higher risk of developing prostate cancer.

5. Exposure to certain chemicals: Men who work with chemicals, such as firefighters or those in the petroleum industry, may be at higher risk of developing prostate cancer.

It's important to note that having one or further of these threat factors doesn't inescapably mean that a man will develop prostate cancer. However, men with these risk factors should be aware of the symptoms of prostate cancer and should talk to their healthcare provider about their risk of the disease.

In summary, prostate cancer is a common type of cancer that affects men. It is often asymptomatic in its early stages, but as cancer progresses, it may cause symptoms such as difficulty urinating, blood in the urine or semen, erectile dysfunction, and pain or discomfort. Men should be aware of these symptoms and should seek medical attention if they persist or worsen over time. Additionally, men with a family history of prostate cancer, who are over the age of 50, or who have other risk factors for the disease should talk to their healthcare provider about their risk and any appropriate screening measures.

How is Prostate Cancer Diagnosed?

Prostate cancer can be diagnosed through several methods, including a digital rectal exam (DRE), a prostate-specific antigen (PSA) blood test, and a prostate biopsy.

During a DRE, a healthcare provider will insert a gloved finger into the rectum to feel for any abnormalities in the prostate gland, such as lumps or hard spots. While this exam can detect some prostate cancers, it is not as effective as other screening methods.

The PSA blood test measures the level of PSA, a protein produced by the prostate gland, in the blood. High levels of PSA can indicate the presence of prostate cancer, but PSA levels can also be elevated for other reasons, such as an enlarged prostate or a urinary tract infection.

If a PSA test indicates an elevated PSA level or a healthcare provider detects abnormalities during a DRE, a prostate biopsy may be recommended. During a biopsy, a small sample of prostate tissue is taken and examined under a microscope for the presence of cancer cells.

It is important to note that not all prostate cancers are detected through screening, and some men may not experience symptoms until the cancer has advanced. Therefore, it is important for men to discuss their risk of prostate cancer with their healthcare provider and to undergo appropriate screening measures as recommended.

Additionally, men who experience any symptoms of prostate cancer, such as difficulty urinating, blood in the urine or semen, or erectile dysfunction, should seek medical attention promptly.

Stages of Prostate Cancer

Prostate cancer is typically classified into four stages, which are determined based on the size and extent of the cancer, as well as whether it has spread to nearby tissues or other parts of the body. These are the following stages of prostate cancer:

Stage I: In this stage, the cancer is confined to the prostate gland and is usually small and slow-growing. It is often detected incidentally during other medical procedures or tests, as there may be no symptoms.

Stage II: At this stage, the cancer is still confined to the prostate gland, but is more advanced than in stage I. The cancer may be larger and growing more quickly, or it may be present in multiple areas of the prostate gland.

Stage III: At this stage, the cancer has spread beyond the prostate gland and may be present in nearby tissues or organs, such as the seminal vesicles or the bladder. It has not yet spread to other parts of the body.

Stage IV: This is the most advanced stage of prostate cancer, and the cancer has spread to other parts of the body, such as the bones or lymph nodes. At this stage, the cancer is often more aggressive and harder to treat.

Determining the stage of prostate cancer is important in developing an appropriate treatment plan. Treatment options for prostate cancer may include watchful waiting or active surveillance for early-stage cancers, surgery, radiation therapy, hormone therapy, chemotherapy, or a combination of these treatments. Your healthcare provider can help you understand the stage of your prostate cancer and work with you to develop a personalized treatment plan.

Types of Prostate Cancer

There are several types of prostate cancer, which can be classified based on the appearance of the cancer cells under a microscope. The most common types of prostate cancer are:

1. Adenocarcinoma This is the most common type of prostate cancer, counting for roughly 95 of all cases. Adenocarcinoma develops from the glandular cells of the prostate gland and typically grows slowly.

2. Small cell carcinoma: This is a rare and aggressive type of prostate cancer that develops from the neuroendocrine cells of the prostate gland. Small cell carcinoma is typically more difficult to treat than adenocarcinoma.

3. Sarcomas: These are rare types of prostate cancer that develop from the connective tissue or

muscle cells in the prostate gland. Sarcomas can be more aggressive than adenocarcinoma and may require more aggressive treatment.

4. Transitional cell carcinoma: This is a rare type of prostate cancer that develops from the cells that line the tubes that carry urine from the bladder through the prostate gland. Transitional cell carcinoma is typically more aggressive than adenocarcinoma.

5. Ductal carcinoma: This is a rare type of prostate cancer that develops from the cells that line the ducts of the prostate gland. Ductal carcinoma can be more aggressive than adenocarcinoma and may require more aggressive treatment.

It is important to note that prostate cancer can also be classified based on how quickly it is growing, as well as whether it has spread beyond the prostate gland. Slow-growing prostate cancers may not require immediate treatment, while faster-growing or more aggressive cancers may require more aggressive treatment. Additionally, prostate cancer can be classified based on the presence or absence of hormone receptors, which can affect treatment options.

The specific type of prostate cancer a person has can affect their treatment options and their prognosis. Your healthcare provider can help you understand the type of prostate cancer you have and work with you to develop an appropriate treatment plan. Regular prostate cancer screening and early detection can help identify the type of cancer and improve the chances of successful treatment.

Chapter 3

Treatment Options: Surgery

Surgery is a common treatment option for prostate cancer, particularly for early-stage cancers that have not spread beyond the prostate gland. The two main types of surgical procedures for prostate cancer are radical prostatectomy and transurethral resection of the prostate (TURP).

Radical prostatectomy involves the surgical removal of the entire prostate gland, as well as the seminal vesicles and some surrounding tissue. The surgery may be performed using traditional open surgery, minimally invasive laparoscopic surgery, or robot-assisted laparoscopic surgery.

Recovery time after radical prostatectomy varies depending on the type of surgery used, but typically involves a hospital stay of several days and several weeks of recovery time at home.

TURP, on the other hand, is a minimally invasive surgical procedure that involves the removal of small pieces of the prostate gland through the urethra. This procedure is typically used to treat urinary symptoms caused by an enlarged prostate but may be used in some cases to remove early-stage prostate cancer.

Recovery time after TURP is typically shorter than after radical prostatectomy, and most patients can go home the same day as the procedure.

While surgery can be an effective treatment option for prostate cancer, it does carry some risks and potential side effects. Common side effects of surgery for prostate cancer include erectile dysfunction, urinary incontinence, and difficulty achieving orgasm.

In some cases, surgery may also damage the nerves that control bladder and bowel function, leading to long-term urinary or bowel problems.

Your healthcare provider can help you understand the risks and benefits of surgery for prostate cancer, as well as help you determine whether surgery is the best treatment option for your case. Other treatment options for prostate cancer may include radiation therapy, hormone therapy, or active surveillance.

Radical Prostatectomy

The surgical procedure that is used to treat localized prostate cancer is Radical Prostatectomy. During this procedure, the entire prostate gland, as well as the seminal vesicles and some surrounding tissue, are removed to eliminate the cancerous cells.

There are several approaches to performing a radical prostatectomy, including open surgery, laparoscopic surgery, and robot-assisted laparoscopic surgery. Open surgery involves making a large incision in the abdomen to access the prostate gland, while laparoscopic surgery uses several small incisions and specialized surgical instruments to remove the prostate gland. Robot-assisted laparoscopic surgery is a type of laparoscopic surgery in which a surgeon uses a robotic system to control the surgical instruments.

Radical prostatectomy is typically recommended for men with early-stage prostate cancer that has not spread beyond the prostate gland. It may also be recommended for men with more advanced prostate cancer that has not responded to other types of treatment.

After a radical prostatectomy, patients typically experience some pain and discomfort and may need to stay in the hospital for several days. Recovery time can vary depending on the type of surgery performed and the individual patient's overall health, but most men can return to their normal activities within some weeks to some months after the procedure.

Like any surgical procedure, radical prostatectomy carries some risks and potential complications. Common side effects of radical prostatectomy include erectile dysfunction, urinary incontinence, and difficulty achieving orgasm. In some cases, the surgery may also damage the nerves that control bladder and bowel function, leading to long-term urinary or bowel problems.

Your healthcare provider can help you understand the risks and benefits of radical prostatectomy, as well as help you determine whether this procedure is the best treatment option for your case. Other treatment options for prostate cancer may include radiation therapy, hormone therapy, or active surveillance.

Robotic-Assisted Laparoscopic Prostatectomy

Robotic-assisted laparoscopic prostatectomy is a minimally invasive surgical procedure used to remove the prostate gland and surrounding tissue to treat localized prostate cancer. During the procedure, a surgeon uses a robotic system to control surgical instruments, which are inserted through small incisions in the abdomen.

The robotic system provides the surgeon with greater precision and control during the procedure, as well as a three-dimensional view of the surgical area. This allows for more precise removal of the prostate gland, with less damage to surrounding tissues and structures.

Robotic-assisted laparoscopic prostatectomy is typically recommended for men with early-stage prostate cancer that has not spread beyond the prostate gland. It may also be recommended for men with more advanced prostate cancer that has not responded to other types of treatment.

After the procedure, patients typically experience some pain and discomfort and may need to stay in the hospital for several days. Recovery time can vary depending on the individual patient's overall health and the extent of the surgery, but most men can return to their normal activities within some weeks to some months after the procedure.

Like any surgical procedure, robotic-assisted laparoscopic prostatectomy carries some risks and potential complications. Common side effects of the procedure include erectile dysfunction, urinary incontinence, and difficulty achieving orgasm. In some cases, the surgery may also damage the nerves that control bladder and bowel function, leading to long-term urinary or bowel problems.

Your healthcare provider can help you understand the risks and benefits of robotic-assisted laparoscopic prostatectomy, as well as help you determine whether this procedure is the best treatment option for your case. Other treatment options for prostate cancer may include radiation therapy, hormone therapy, or active surveillance.

Radiation Therapy

Radiation therapy is a treatment for prostate cancer that uses high-energy radiation to kill cancer cells. The radiation can be delivered either externally or internally.

External radiation therapy, also called external beam radiation therapy, uses a machine outside the body to deliver radiation to the prostate gland. The radiation is carefully targeted to the prostate gland, and the surrounding tissues and organs are protected as much as possible. Treatment is generally given in diurnal sessions over several weeks.

Internal radiation therapy, also called brachytherapy, involves placing tiny radioactive seeds directly into the prostate gland. The seeds emit radiation for several weeks to several months, depending on the type of seed used. The radiation is carefully targeted to the prostate gland, and the surrounding tissues and organs are protected as much as possible.

Radiation therapy may be recommended for men with localized prostate cancer, as well as for men with more advanced prostate cancer that has spread to nearby tissues or organs. Radiation therapy may also be used as a follow-up treatment after surgery.

After radiation therapy, patients may experience some side effects, including fatigue, skin irritation, and urinary or bowel problems. These side effects are generally temporary and can be managed with specifics and other treatments.

Like any treatment for prostate cancer, radiation therapy carries some risks and potential complications. In rare cases, radiation therapy may cause long-term damage to nearby tissues or organs or may increase the risk of developing secondary cancer.

Your healthcare provider can help you understand the risks and benefits of radiation therapy, as well as help you determine whether this treatment is the best option for your case.

Other treatment options for prostate cancer may include surgery, hormone therapy, or active surveillance.

External Beam Radiation Therapy

External beam radiation therapy (EBRT) is a type of radiation therapy that uses high-energy X-rays or other types of radiation to kill cancer cells in the prostate gland. During the procedure, a machine called a linear accelerator delivers radiation beams to the prostate gland from outside the body.

The radiation is carefully targeted to the prostate gland while minimizing exposure to surrounding tissues and organs.

EBRT is typically delivered in daily sessions over several weeks. The treatment schedule and duration will depend on the individual case and the stage of the cancer.

EBRT is usually recommended for men with early-stage prostate cancer, as well as for men with more advanced prostate cancer that has not spread beyond the prostate gland. External beam radiation therapy may also be used as a follow-up treatment after surgery.

After EBRT, patients may experience some side effects, including fatigue, skin irritation, and urinary or bowel problems. These side effects are generally temporary and can be managed with specifics and other treatments.

Like any treatment for prostate cancer, EBRT carries some risks and potential complications. In rare cases, EBRT may cause long-term damage to nearby tissues or organs or may increase the risk of developing secondary cancer.

Your healthcare provider can help you understand the risks and benefits of EBRT, as well as help you determine whether this treatment is the best option for your case. Other treatment options for prostate cancer may include surgery, hormone therapy, or active surveillance.

Brachytherapy (Seed Implants)

Brachytherapy, also known as seed implantation, is a type of radiation therapy that involves placing small radioactive seeds directly into the prostate gland. The seeds emit radiation for several weeks to several months, depending on the type of seed used. The radiation is carefully targeted to the prostate gland while minimizing exposure to surrounding tissues and organs.

Brachytherapy is typically recommended for men with early-stage prostate cancer, as well as for men with intermediate-risk prostate cancer. It may also be used as a boost therapy after external beam radiation therapy.

The procedure is typically done under anesthesia and involves placing the seeds directly into the prostate gland using small needles. The number and placement of seeds will depend on the individual case and the stage of the cancer.

After brachytherapy, patients may experience some side effects, including urinary problems and bowel problems. These side effects are generally temporary and can be managed with specifics and other treatments.

Like any treatment for prostate cancer, brachytherapy carries some risks and potential complications. In rare cases, brachytherapy may cause long-term damage to nearby tissues or organs or may increase the risk of developing secondary cancer.

Your healthcare provider can help you understand the risks and benefits of brachytherapy, as well as help you determine whether this treatment is the best option for your case. Other treatment options for prostate cancer may include surgery, external beam radiation therapy, hormone therapy, or active surveillance.

Hormone Therapy

Hormone therapy, also known as androgen deprivation therapy (ADT), is a treatment for prostate cancer that involves reducing the levels of male hormones (androgens) in the body, particularly testosterone. Androgens can stimulate the growth of prostate cancer cells, so reducing their levels can slow the growth of cancer and shrink the prostate gland.

Hormone therapy is typically used for men with advanced prostate cancer or for men with intermediate-risk prostate cancer who are not candidates for surgery or radiation therapy. It may also be used in combination with other treatments, such as radiation therapy or chemotherapy.

Hormone therapy can be delivered in several ways, including through injections, pills, or implants. The treatment may be temporary or ongoing, depending on the individual case and the stage of the cancer.

Hormone therapy can have side effects, including fatigue, decreased libido, hot flashes, weight gain, and loss of muscle mass. These side effects can often be managed with medications and other treatments.

Hormone therapy can also increase the risk of developing osteoporosis and may increase the risk of cardiovascular disease. Regular monitoring and follow-up with a healthcare provider are important to manage these potential risks.

While hormone therapy can slow the growth of prostate cancer and improve symptoms, it is not a cure for prostate cancer. Over time, some prostate cancer cells may become resistant to hormone therapy, leading to the need for other treatments.

Androgen Deprivation Therapy (ADT)

Androgen deprivation therapy (ADT), also known as hormone therapy, is a type of treatment for prostate cancer that works by reducing the levels of androgens, particularly testosterone, in the body. Androgens can stimulate the growth of prostate cancer cells, so reducing their levels can slow the growth of cancer and shrink the prostate gland.

ADT can be delivered in several ways, including through injections, pills, or implants. The treatment may be temporary or ongoing, depending on the individual case and the stage of the cancer.

ADT is typically used for men with advanced prostate cancer or for men with intermediate-risk prostate cancer who are not candidates for surgery or radiation therapy. It may also be used in combination with other treatments, such as radiation therapy or chemotherapy.

ADT can have side effects, including fatigue, decreased libido, hot flashes, weight gain, and loss of muscle mass. These side effects can often be managed with medications and other treatments.

ADT can also increase the risk of developing osteoporosis and may increase the risk of cardiovascular disease. Regular monitoring and follow-up with a healthcare provider are important to manage these potential risks.

While ADT can slow the growth of prostate cancer and improve symptoms, it is not a cure for prostate cancer. Over time, some prostate cancer cells may become resistant to ADT, leading to the need for other treatments.

Chemotherapy

Chemotherapy is a type of cancer treatment that uses drugs to kill rapidly dividing cells, including cancer cells. Chemotherapy is typically used for men with advanced or metastatic prostate cancer that has spread beyond the prostate gland.

Chemotherapy for prostate cancer is usually given in cycles, with a period of treatment followed by a period of rest. The drugs used in chemotherapy for prostate cancer can be given intravenously (through an IV) or orally (in pill form).

Chemotherapy can have side effects, including nausea, vomiting, fatigue, hair loss, and an increased risk of infections. These side effects can often be managed with medications and other treatments.

Chemotherapy can also damage healthy cells in the body, leading to potential long-term side effects. Regular monitoring and follow-up with a healthcare provider are important to manage these potential risks.

While chemotherapy can slow the growth of prostate cancer and improve symptoms, it is not a cure for prostate cancer. Chemotherapy is often used in combination with other treatments, such as hormone therapy or radiation therapy, to improve outcomes for men with advanced prostate cancer.

Watchful Waiting or Active Surveillance

Watchful waiting or active surveillance is a management approach for men with low-risk or very low-risk prostate cancer. This approach involves closely monitoring the cancer with regular check-ups and tests, but not treating the cancer immediately.

Watchful waiting is typically recommended for older men or men with other medical conditions that may make treatment more difficult. Active surveillance is typically recommended for younger men with low-risk prostate cancer who are concerned about the potential side effects of treatment.

During watchful waiting or active surveillance, men will have regular prostate-specific antigen (PSA) tests and digital rectal exams (DREs) to monitor the progression of cancer. If the cancer starts to grow or become more aggressive, treatment may be recommended.

Watchful waiting and active surveillance can have psychological benefits for men who may be worried about the potential side effects of treatment, such as incontinence or impotence.

However, it is important to have regular check-ups and follow-ups with a healthcare provider to monitor the cancer and ensure that treatment is initiated if necessary. Watchful waiting and active surveillance are not appropriate for all men with prostate cancer.

Men with high-risk or aggressive prostate cancer are typically recommended to receive immediate treatment, such as surgery or radiation therapy. It is important to discuss all treatment options with a healthcare provider to determine the best course of action for individual cases.

Clinical Trials

Clinical trials are research studies that are designed to evaluate the safety and effectiveness of new treatments for prostate cancer. These studies are typically conducted in phases, with each phase designed to answer specific questions about the new treatment.

Phase I trials are generally the first step in testing a new treatment. These trials are designed to determine the safety and dosing of the new treatment.

Phase II trials are designed to evaluate the effectiveness of the new treatment in a small group of patients. These trials also evaluate the side effects of the treatment and determine the appropriate dosing.

Phase III trials are large-scale studies that compare the new treatment to the current standard of care. These trials are designed to determine whether the new treatment is more effective than the current standard of care.

Clinical trials can have many benefits for men with prostate cancer. They may provide access to new treatments that are not yet available to the general public, and they may also provide additional monitoring and follow-up care.

However, clinical trials also carry some risks. The new treatment may not be effective, and there may be unknown risks associated with the treatment. Men need to discuss the potential benefits and risks of participating in a clinical trial with their healthcare provider.

Participation in clinical trials is typically voluntary. Men who are interested in participating in a clinical trial should discuss their options with their healthcare provider and carefully consider the potential benefits and risks before making a decision.

Chapter 4

Coping with Treatment Side Effects

Prostate cancer treatment can have a variety of side effects, including fatigue, nausea, hair loss, incontinence, and impotence. Coping with these side effects can be challenging, but there are strategies that men can use to manage them.

The common side effect of prostate cancer treatment is Fatigue. Men can manage fatigue by getting plenty of rest, eating a healthy diet, and engaging in light exercise.

Nausea can be managed by eating small, frequent meals throughout the day and avoiding foods that are high in fat or spicy. Some men may also benefit from anti-nausea medications.

Hair loss is a side effect of chemotherapy. Men can manage hair loss by using gentle shampoos and avoiding harsh chemicals or heat styling tools. Wearing a wig or hat can also help to conceal hair loss.

Incontinence is a common side effect of surgery or radiation therapy. Men can manage incontinence by doing Kegel exercises to strengthen the pelvic floor muscles. Using pads or other absorbent products can also help to manage urinary leakage.

Impotence is a potential side effect of surgery or radiation therapy. Men can manage impotence by using medications such as sildenafil (Viagra) or tadalafil (Cialis) to improve erectile function. Other options include penile injections, vacuum devices, or penile implants.

Counseling or support groups can also be helpful for men who are coping with the side effects of prostate cancer treatment. These resources can provide emotional support and practical advice for managing side effects.

Men need to discuss any side effects they are experiencing with their healthcare provider. In some cases, changes to the treatment plan or medication adjustments may be necessary to manage side effects effectively.

Common Side Effects of Prostate Cancer Treatment: Urinary Incontinence

Urinary incontinence is a potential side effect of prostate cancer treatment, particularly after surgery or radiation therapy. It occurs when a man loses control over his bladder and leaks urine involuntarily. Urinary incontinence can be a source of embarrassment and affect a man's quality of life, but some strategies can help to manage this condition.

One of the most effective ways to manage urinary incontinence is through Kegel exercises. These exercises involve contracting and relaxing the muscles in the pelvic floor, which can help to improve bladder control. Men can perform

Kegel exercises several times a day, starting with a few repetitions and gradually increasing the number over time.

Another strategy for managing urinary incontinence is to use absorbent pads or adult diapers. These products can help to prevent leaks and provide a sense of security for men who are experiencing incontinence. There are many different types of pads and diapers available, and men can choose the product that best meets their needs.

Men can also manage urinary incontinence by modifying their fluid intake. Drinking less fluids before bedtime or when going out can help to reduce the frequency of urination and prevent accidents. Avoiding beverages that can irritate the bladder, such as alcohol and caffeine, can also be helpful.

In some cases, medication may be prescribed to help manage urinary incontinence. These medications can help to relax the bladder or strengthen the muscles that control urination. Your healthcare provider can determine if medication is appropriate and recommend a suitable treatment plan.

Men need to discuss any symptoms of urinary incontinence with their healthcare provider. Your provider can assess the severity of incontinence and recommend appropriate treatment options. With proper management, many men can successfully manage urinary incontinence and maintain a good quality of life.

Erectile Dysfunction

Erectile dysfunction, also known as impotence, is another potential side effect of prostate cancer treatment. It occurs when a man has difficulty achieving or maintaining an erection sufficient for sexual activity. Erectile dysfunction can be a distressing and frustrating experience for men, but some strategies can help to manage this condition.

One of the most effective ways to manage erectile dysfunction is through the use of oral medications, such as sildenafil (Viagra), tadalafil (Cialis), and vardenafil (Levitra). These medications work by increasing blood flow to the penis, which can help to improve erectile function. These medications are typically prescribed by a healthcare provider and should be used as directed.

Another strategy for managing erectile dysfunction is through the use of vacuum erection devices (VEDs). These devices consist of a plastic tube that is placed over the penis and a hand pump that creates a vacuum to draw blood into the penis. Once an erection is achieved, a ring is placed at the base of the penis to maintain the erection.

In some cases, injection therapy may be recommended to manage erectile dysfunction. This involves the injection of medication directly into the penis, which can help to increase blood flow and improve erectile function. This treatment is typically administered by a healthcare provider.

Penile implants are another option for managing erectile dysfunction. These devices are surgically implanted into the penis and can be inflated to create an erection. Penile implants are typically reserved for men who have not had success with other treatments.

Men need to discuss any symptoms of erectile dysfunction with their healthcare provider. Your provider can assess the severity of erectile dysfunction and recommend appropriate treatment options. With proper management, many men can successfully manage erectile dysfunction and maintain a satisfying sex life.

Hot Flashes

Hot flashes are a common side effect of hormone therapy used to treat prostate cancer. Hormone therapy works by reducing the levels of testosterone in the body, which can help to slow the growth and spread of prostate cancer. However, this reduction in testosterone can also cause hot flashes, which are characterized by sudden feelings of warmth, sweating, and flushing of the skin.

While hot flashes can be uncomfortable and disruptive, some strategies can help to manage this side effect. One of the most effective ways to manage hot flashes is through lifestyle changes. This may include avoiding triggers such as hot beverages, spicy foods, and alcohol, and dressing in layers to easily remove clothing during a hot flash.

Exercise may also help manage hot flashes. Studies have shown that regular physical activity can reduce the frequency and severity of hot flashes in men undergoing hormone therapy for prostate cancer. Exercise can also have other health benefits such as reducing stress and improving overall mood.

In some cases, medication may be recommended to manage hot flashes. Antidepressants such as venlafaxine and paroxetine are effective in reducing the frequency and severity of hot flashes in men undergoing hormone therapy for prostate cancer. Other medications such as gabapentin and clonidine may also be used to manage hot flashes.

It is important for men undergoing hormone therapy to discuss any symptoms of hot flashes with their healthcare provider. Your provider can assess the severity of hot flashes and recommend appropriate treatment options. With proper management, many men can successfully manage hot flashes and maintain a good quality of life while undergoing prostate cancer treatment.

Tips for Managing Side Effects

Managing the side effects of prostate cancer treatment can be challenging, but some strategies can help. Here are some tips for managing common side effects:

1. Communicate with your healthcare team: It is important to keep your healthcare team informed about any side effects you are experiencing. They can offer suggestions and recommend treatment options to help manage symptoms.

2. Follow a healthy diet: Eating a healthy diet can help reduce side effects such as fatigue and nausea. It's important to eat a balanced diet that includes a plenitude of fruits, vegetables, whole grains, and spare proteins.

3. Stay hydrated: Drinking plenty of water can help reduce side effects such as constipation and dehydration. It's important to stay doused throughout the day by drinking water and other fluids.

4. Get enough rest: Rest is important for managing side effects such as fatigue. Make sure

to get enough sleep each night and take breaks throughout the day to rest and recharge.

5. Exercise regularly: Exercise can help reduce side effects such as fatigue and improve overall mood. It is important to talk to your doctor before starting any exercise program.

6. Manage stress: Stress can exacerbate side effects and impact overall well-being. Consider rehearsing relaxation ways similar to deep breathing, contemplation, or yoga to help manage stress.

7. Seek support: Talking to family, friends, or a support group can help manage side effects and cope with the emotional impact of prostate cancer treatment.

It is important to remember that managing side effects is an ongoing process that may require adjustments over time. By working closely with your healthcare team and making lifestyle changes, it is possible to effectively manage side effects and maintain a good quality of life during and after prostate cancer treatment.

Alternative and Complementary Therapies

Alternative and complementary therapies are often used alongside traditional medical treatments for prostate cancer. These therapies are not intended to replace medical treatments, but rather to supplement them and help manage side effects. Here are some common alternative and complementary therapies used in prostate cancer treatment:

1. Acupuncture: This traditional Chinese medicine involves the use of thin needles inserted at specific points on the body to alleviate pain and other symptoms.

2. Massage therapy: Massage can help reduce stress and anxiety, alleviate pain, and improve overall well-being.

3. Herbal remedies: Some herbs such as saw palmetto and green tea are believed to have anti-inflammatory and antioxidant properties that may help reduce prostate cancer risk and improve outcomes.

4. Mind-body techniques: Practices such as meditation, yoga, and tai chi can help reduce stress and improve overall well-being.

5. Nutritional supplements: Some supplements such as vitamin D and omega-3 fatty acids are believed to have potential health benefits for prostate cancer patients.

It is important to discuss any alternative or complementary therapies with your healthcare provider before starting them, as some may interact with medications or have potential risks.

Additionally, some alternative therapies may not be backed by scientific evidence and should be used with caution. While alternative and complementary therapies may help manage side effects and improve overall well-being, they should not be used as a substitute for traditional medical treatments.

It is important to work closely with your healthcare team to develop a comprehensive treatment plan that includes both medical and complementary therapies to effectively manage prostate cancer and its side effects.

Chapter 5

Lifestyle Changes for a Healthy Recovery: Nutrition and Diet

Nutrition and diet play an important role in prostate cancer treatment and recovery. Here are some tips for maintaining a healthy diet during prostate cancer treatment:

1. Focus on whole foods: Eating a diet that is rich in fruits, vegetables, whole grains, and lean proteins can help provide your body with the nutrients it needs to support healing and overall health.

2. Limit red meat and processed foods: Red meat and processed foods have been linked to an increased risk of prostate cancer. Try to limit your intake of these foods and choose lean proteins like chicken, fish, and tofu instead.

3. Incorporate healthy fats: Omega-3 fatty acids found in fish, nuts, and seeds can help reduce

inflammation in the body and support overall health. Additionally, monounsaturated fats found in foods like avocado, olive oil, and nuts can help improve heart health.

4. Stay hydrated: Drinking plenty of water can help flush toxins from your body and support overall health.

5. Consider supplements: Certain supplements, such as vitamin D and selenium, may have potential health benefits for prostate cancer patients. However, it is important to discuss any supplements with your healthcare provider before starting them, as some may interact with medications or have potential risks.

It is also important to maintain a healthy weight during prostate cancer treatment. Being overweight or obese has been linked to an increased risk of prostate cancer recurrence and can also increase the risk of other health complications. Eating a healthy diet and getting regular exercise can help you maintain a healthy weight and support overall health during and after prostate cancer treatment.

Remember to discuss any dietary changes with your healthcare provider before making them. They can guide the best diet and nutrition plan for your individual needs and help you navigate any potential interactions with medications or treatments.

Exercise and Physical Activity

Exercise and physical activity are important components of prostate cancer treatment and recovery. Here are some tips for incorporating physical activity into your routine during and after treatment:

1. Start slow: It is important to start slow and gradually increase your activity level, especially if you have been inactive or are recovering from surgery or other treatments. Begin with low-intensity activities like walking, stretching, or light resistance training.

2. Aim for at least 150 minutes of moderate exercise per week: The American Cancer Society recommends that cancer survivors aim for at least 150 minutes of moderate exercise per week. This includes activities like brisk walking, cycling, swimming, or dancing.

3. Incorporate strength training: Strength training can help improve muscle mass and bone density, which can be particularly important for older adults or those undergoing hormone therapy. Consider incorporating exercises like push-ups, lunges, or using resistance bands.

4. Listen to your body: It is necessary to listen to your body and not push yourself too hard. If you are experiencing fatigue or other symptoms, it is okay to take a break or modify your activity level.

5. Consider working with a physical therapist: A physical therapist can provide guidance on safe exercises and modifications that may be

necessary depending on your treatment plan and individual needs.

In addition to the physical benefits, regular exercise can also provide emotional and psychological benefits, such as reducing stress and improving mood. It is important to discuss any exercise plans with your healthcare provider, particularly if you have any physical limitations or medical concerns. They can guide the best exercise plan for your individual needs and help you stay safe during your recovery.

Stress Management and Relaxation Techniques

Prostate cancer can be a stressful and challenging experience, and managing stress is an important part of coping with the disease. Here are some stress management and relaxation techniques that may be helpful for prostate cancer patients:

1. Mindfulness meditation: Mindfulness meditation involves focusing on the present moment and observing thoughts and sensations without judgment. This practice has been shown to reduce stress and improve mental health.

2. Deep breathing: Taking slow, deep breaths can help reduce stress and promote relaxation. Try inhaling deeply through the nose for a count of four, holding the breath for a count of seven, and exhaling slowly through the mouth for a count of eight.

3. Progressive muscle relaxation: This technique involves tensing and relaxing different muscle groups in the body, starting at the feet and working up to the head. This can help in reducing tension and promote relaxation.

4. Yoga: Yoga combines physical movement with mindfulness and breathing techniques, making it a potentially effective stress management tool. Many yoga studios and online

platforms offer classes tailored specifically for cancer patients.

5. Tai chi: This gentle form of exercise involves slow, flowing movements and deep breathing, and has been shown to reduce stress and improve overall well-being.

6. Guided imagery: This technique involves visualizing peaceful and calming scenes or experiences to reduce stress and promote relaxation. Guided imagery can be done with the help of a trained professional or through audio recordings.

In addition to these techniques, it can be helpful to identify and address sources of stress in your life, such as financial concerns or relationship problems. Talk therapy or support groups may also help manage stress and emotional well-being during prostate cancer treatment.

Sleep and Rest

Getting enough rest and sleep is important for overall health and well-being, especially when going through prostate cancer treatment. Here are some tips for getting quality sleep and rest during this time:

1. Stick to a regular sleep schedule: Go to bed and wake up at the same time every day, even during weekends.

2. Create a comfortable sleep environment: Make sure your bedroom is cool, quiet, and dark. Make use of a comfortable mattress and pillows.

3. Limit screen time before bed: The blue light emitted by electronic devices can interfere with sleep. Avoid screens for at least an hour before bedtime.

4. Avoid taking caffeine and alcohol: Both caffeine and alcohol can disrupt sleep. Avoid

these substances, especially in the hours leading up to bedtime.

5. Incorporate relaxation techniques: The stress of prostate cancer treatment can make it difficult to fall and stay asleep. Try incorporating relaxation techniques such as deep breathing, guided imagery, or progressive muscle relaxation before bedtime.

6. Take naps if needed: It's okay to take short naps during the day if you're feeling tired. Just make sure to keep them short (20-30 minutes) and earlier in the day to avoid interfering with nighttime sleep.

7. Talk to your doctor: If you're having trouble sleeping despite trying these strategies, talk to your doctor. They may be able to recommend additional strategies or medication to help you sleep better.

Getting enough rest and sleep can help you feel more energized and better able to cope with the challenges of prostate cancer treatment. It's important to prioritize self-care during this time, and that includes making sure you're getting enough rest and sleep.

Smoking Cessation and Alcohol Moderation

Quitting smoking and moderating alcohol consumption are important steps for overall health, especially during prostate cancer treatment. Here's why:

Smoking can increase the risk of prostate cancer recurrence and decrease the effectiveness of treatment. Smoking can also cause other health problems such as lung cancer, heart disease, and stroke.

Quitting smoking can improve overall health, reduce the risk of cancer recurrence, and improve the effectiveness of treatment. Alcohol consumption, especially in excess, can also increase the risk of prostate cancer recurrence and cause other health problems such as liver disease and high blood pressure. Moderation is key - it's recommended to limit alcohol intake to no more than one drink per day for men.

If you're struggling with smoking cessation or alcohol moderation, here are some tips to help:

1. Talk to your doctor: Your doctor can provide resources and support to help you quit smoking or moderate alcohol consumption.

2. Seek support: Join a support group or talk to a counselor to help you stay motivated and accountable.

3. Identify triggers: Understand what triggers your smoking or drinking behavior and develop strategies to cope with these triggers.

4. Find healthy alternatives: Replace smoking or drinking with healthy alternatives such as exercise, meditation, or hobbies.

5. Set goals: Set realistic goals and track your progress to stay motivated.

6. Be patient and persistent: Quitting smoking or moderating alcohol consumption can be challenging. Don't give up - keep trying and seek help when needed.

Making these lifestyle changes can be difficult, but the benefits to overall health and cancer treatment outcomes are significant. Talk to your doctor about how you can make these changes and get the support you need.

Chapter 6

Emotional Support and Coping Strategies: Understanding the Emotional Impact of Prostate Cancer

Prostate cancer not only affects the physical health of a person, but it can also take a toll on their emotional well-being. A diagnosis of cancer can cause feelings of fear, anxiety, and depression. It is important to recognize and address the emotional impact of prostate cancer to cope effectively with the disease.

Fear and anxiety are common emotions that people experience after being diagnosed with prostate cancer. Fear can be caused by uncertainty about the future, concerns about treatment, and the possibility of the cancer returning.

Anxiety can also be a result of these uncertainties, as well as the stress of undergoing medical tests and treatments. It is important to communicate with healthcare providers and loved ones about these feelings and concerns.

Depression is another common emotional response to a cancer diagnosis. It can be caused by the stress of the illness and its treatment, as well as changes in physical appearance and function. Depression can also make it more difficult to cope with treatment and manage symptoms.

It is important to seek help from a mental health professional or counselor if feelings of depression persist. Social support can be a key factor in coping with the emotional impact of prostate cancer. Talking to family members, friends, or a support group can help alleviate feelings of loneliness and isolation.

Support groups can also provide helpful information about coping strategies and resources for dealing with the disease.

In addition to seeking social support, self-care is an important aspect of managing the emotional impact of prostate cancer. This can include engaging in relaxing activities such as meditation or yoga, pursuing hobbies or interests, and maintaining a healthy lifestyle through exercise and diet.

It is important to remember that the emotional impact of prostate cancer is normal and valid. Seeking support from loved ones and healthcare providers, practicing self-care, and staying informed about the disease and treatment options can help manage the emotional impact of prostate cancer.

Coping with Anxiety and Depression

Being diagnosed with prostate cancer can be a stressful and overwhelming experience, which can lead to anxiety and depression. Coping with these emotional challenges can be just as important as treating the physical aspects of the disease.

It is normal to experience a range of emotions, such as fear, anger, sadness, and confusion, and it is essential to have a support system to help manage these feelings. One of the best ways to manage anxiety and depression is to talk to someone.

Sharing your feelings with family, friends, or a professional counselor can help you process your emotions and develop coping strategies. Many cancer centers offer counseling and support groups specifically for cancer patients and their families.

In addition to seeking professional help, there are also self-care techniques that can help manage anxiety and depression. These include:

- Exercise: Endorphins are released by exercise, which is natural mood boosters. Even light exercise such as walking can help reduce stress and anxiety.

- Mindfulness: Mindfulness practices such as meditation, deep breathing, and yoga can help reduce stress and promote relaxation.

- Hobbies: Engaging in hobbies and activities you enjoy can provide a sense of purpose and help distract from negative thoughts.

- Positive self-talk: It can be easy to fall into negative self-talk, but focusing on positive thoughts and affirmations can help improve mood and outlook.

- Social support: Spending time with loved ones and friends can provide emotional support and help reduce feelings of isolation.

It is essential to be patient and kind to yourself as you navigate the emotional impact of prostate cancer. Remember that it is normal to have good and bad days, and seeking help is a sign of strength, not weakness.

Building a Support System

A prostate cancer diagnosis can be overwhelming and stressful, which is why it's important to have a strong support system in place. This can include family, friends, healthcare professionals, support groups, and online communities. The tips for building a support system are:

1. Communicate with your loved ones: It's important to be open and honest with your family and friends about your diagnosis and

treatment plan. Let them know how they can support you and what you need from them.

2. Join a support group: Support groups can be a great source of comfort and information. They provide an opportunity to connect with others who are going through a similar experience and can offer valuable advice and support.

3. Talk to a therapist: It's common to experience anxiety, depression, and other emotional challenges when dealing with cancer. A therapist can help you process your emotions and develop coping strategies.

4. Connect with online communities: There are many online communities and forums dedicated to prostate cancer where you can connect with others, share your experiences, and ask questions.

5. Stay involved in your treatment: It's important to stay involved in your treatment plan and be an

active participant in your healthcare. It will help you feel more in control and empowered.

Building a support system takes time and effort, but it can be a valuable source of comfort and strength during your prostate cancer journey. Remember that it's okay to ask for help and lean on others during this challenging time.

Support Groups and Counseling

Receiving a diagnosis of prostate cancer can be overwhelming and emotionally challenging. It is common for patients to experience anxiety, depression, fear, and uncertainty about the future. Coping with these emotions and managing the challenges of treatment can be challenging, but it is important to remember that you do not have to face these challenges alone.

Support groups and counseling can be beneficial for those with prostate cancer. These resources offer an opportunity to connect with others who are going through similar experiences and to gain insight and guidance from professionals who specialize in cancer care.

Support groups can provide emotional support and practical advice on managing treatment side effects, navigating the healthcare system, and coping with the emotional impact of the disease. They can also offer a sense of community and help patients feel less isolated.

There are a variety of support groups available, including those that are specifically tailored to men with prostate cancer, as well as general cancer support groups. Counseling is another helpful resource for managing the emotional impact of prostate cancer.

Mental health professionals can offer a safe and confidential space to talk about fears, concerns, and emotional struggles related to the disease. They can also help patients develop coping strategies, manage stress, and address any underlying mental health concerns, such as anxiety or depression.

Counseling can be provided in a variety of settings, including individual therapy, family therapy, or couples therapy. Some cancer centers may also offer specialized counseling services, such as cognitive-behavioral therapy or mindfulness-based stress reduction.

It is important to remember that seeking support and counseling is a sign of strength, not weakness. Receiving a prostate cancer diagnosis can be overwhelming, and it is natural to feel a range of emotions.

However, with the help of a supportive community and mental health professionals, patients can develop effective coping strategies, manage their emotions, and navigate the challenges of treatment with greater ease.

Chapter 7

Follow-Up Care and Surveillance: Monitoring for Recurrence

Monitoring for recurrence is a crucial aspect of prostate cancer survivorship. Even after successful treatment, there is a chance that prostate cancer may recur. Therefore, regular follow-up care is important to detect any recurrence early and begin treatment promptly.

The frequency of follow-up visits and tests may vary depending on the stage of cancer, type of treatment, and individual patient factors. Generally, follow-up visits are scheduled every 3-6 months for the first few years after treatment, and then less frequently over time if there is no evidence of recurrence.

During follow-up visits, a healthcare provider may perform a physical exam and order blood tests, such as prostate-specific antigen (PSA) tests, to monitor for any signs of recurrence.

PSA is a protein produced by the prostate gland, and levels of PSA in the blood may rise if prostate cancer recurs. Imaging tests, such as bone scans or CT scans, may also be ordered if there is a suspicion of recurrence.

If a recurrence is detected, treatment options will depend on the extent and location of the recurrence, as well as the patient's overall health and treatment history. Treatment may include additional surgery, radiation therapy, hormone therapy, chemotherapy, or a combination of these therapies.

Prostate cancer survivors need to be aware of the signs and symptoms of recurrence, such as difficulty urinating, blood in the urine or semen, bone pain, or unexplained weight loss. Any new or concerning symptoms should be reported to a healthcare provider right away for evaluation.

In addition to regular follow-up care, prostate cancer survivors can take steps to reduce their risk of recurrence. This includes maintaining a healthy lifestyle, such as eating a nutritious diet, exercising regularly, and avoiding tobacco and excessive alcohol consumption. It is also important to manage any ongoing side effects of treatment, as these may affect the quality of life and adherence to follow-up care.

Overall, monitoring for recurrence is an essential part of prostate cancer survivorship. With regular follow-up care and a healthy lifestyle, prostate cancer survivors can reduce their risk of recurrence and live long, fulfilling lives.

Prostate-Specific Antigen (PSA) Testing

Prostate-specific antigen (PSA) testing is a blood test used to detect prostate cancer and monitor its progression. The test measures the amount of PSA, a protein produced by the prostate gland, in the blood. Elevated levels of PSA may indicate the presence of cancer or other prostate conditions, such as inflammation or enlargement of the gland.

PSA testing is not a perfect diagnostic tool, as some men with high levels of PSA do not have prostate cancer, while others with low levels of PSA do have the disease. However, when used in combination with other diagnostic tests, such as a digital rectal exam (DRE) and a biopsy, PSA testing can help identify men who may benefit from further evaluation or treatment.

The American Cancer Society recommends that men discuss the benefits and risks of PSA testing with their healthcare provider, starting at age 50 for most men, or earlier for those at higher risk, such as African American men or men with a family history of prostate cancer.

The decision to have PSA testing should be based on an individual's personal risk factors, such as age, family history, and overall health, as well as their preferences and values. If prostate cancer is diagnosed, PSA testing can be used to monitor the effectiveness of treatment and detect any signs of recurrence.

PSA levels may rise after treatment due to the presence of residual cancer cells or recurrent disease. Regular PSA testing, along with other monitoring methods such as imaging tests and physical exams, can help detect recurrence early and guide decisions about further treatment.

It is important to note that PSA testing alone should not be used to make treatment decisions for prostate cancer. The stage and grade of the cancer, as well as the patient's overall health and other factors, must also be taken into consideration. Patients should discuss their cases with their healthcare provider to determine the best course of treatment and monitoring.

Imaging Tests

Imaging tests are commonly used to monitor for prostate cancer recurrence. These tests use various technologies to create detailed images of the inside of the body, allowing doctors to see if the cancer has spread or come back.

One common imaging test is a bone scan, which is used to detect cancer that has spread to the bones. During a bone scan, a small amount of radioactive material is injected into a vein, and then a special camera is used to take pictures of the bones. Areas, where the material accumulates, can indicate the presence of cancer.

Another imaging test commonly used for prostate cancer is a computed tomography (CT) scan. This test uses X-rays and a computer to create detailed images of the body. CT scans can be used to look for cancer that has spread to nearby lymph nodes or other organs.

Magnetic resonance imaging (MRI) is another imaging test that can be used to monitor prostate cancer recurrence. MRI uses important attractions and radio swells to produce detailed images of the body. It can be used to look for cancer that has spread to the bones or other organs.

Positron emission tomography (PET) scans are a newer type of imaging test that can be used to monitor prostate cancer recurrence. During a PET scan, a small amount of radioactive material is injected into a vein, and then a special camera is used to create images of the body. This test can be used to look for cancer that has spread to distant organs.

In some cases, a combination of imaging tests may be used to monitor for prostate cancer recurrence. The choice of tests or tests used will depend on the individual case and the specific needs of the patient. Regular monitoring and testing are important for detecting any recurrence of prostate cancer early, when treatment options may be more effective.

Understanding Test Results

Understanding test results is an important aspect of monitoring for prostate cancer recurrence. There are several tests that doctors use to determine if the cancer has returned after treatment. The two main tests are the prostate-specific antigen (PSA) test and imaging tests.

PSA testing is done by taking a blood sample and measuring the level of PSA, a protein produced by the prostate gland. If the PSA level rises after treatment, it can be an indication that the cancer has come back. However, it's important to note that PSA levels can also rise for other reasons, such as an enlarged prostate or an infection.

Imaging tests are used to look for signs of cancer in the body. The most common imaging tests used for prostate cancer are bone scans, CT scans, and MRI scans. Bone scans can detect cancer that has spread to the bones, while CT scans and MRI scans can show if the cancer has spread to other organs or tissues.

Once the tests are done, it's important to understand the results. If the PSA level rises or there are signs of cancer on imaging tests, it doesn't necessarily mean that treatment is needed right away. Doctors may recommend monitoring the situation with more frequent testing or additional imaging tests to determine if the cancer is growing or if it's slow-growing cancer that may not need immediate treatment.

Patients need to discuss test results with their doctors and ask any questions they may have. Understanding the results and what they mean can help patients make informed decisions about their care and treatment options. It's also important for patients to keep track of their test results and bring them to all appointments so that doctors have a complete picture of their health history.

Chapter 8

Advocacy and Education: Advocating for Yourself and Others

Advocacy is an important aspect of the prostate cancer journey, not just for oneself, but also for others who are affected by the disease. Advocacy involves speaking up for oneself or others, promoting awareness of the disease, and influencing changes in policies or practices to improve the lives of those affected by prostate cancer.

One of the most important ways to advocate for oneself or others is by becoming informed about the disease and its management. It is important to understand the latest treatment options and to work with healthcare providers to develop a personalized treatment plan.

It is also important to understand the potential side effects of treatment and to be aware of strategies for managing them. Advocacy can also involve promoting awareness of prostate cancer in the community. This can include participating in fundraising events for prostate cancer research, promoting prostate cancer screening and early detection, and sharing one's personal story to inspire others.

Another important aspect of advocacy is influencing policy and practice changes that affect the lives of those affected by prostate cancer. This can include advocating for increased funding for prostate cancer research, promoting policies that ensure access to affordable and high-quality healthcare, and working to eliminate disparities in prostate cancer care.

Advocacy also involves being an active participant in one's care. This means asking questions, sharing concerns, and working collaboratively with healthcare providers to make informed decisions about treatment options. It also means being an active participant in ongoing monitoring for recurrence and taking steps to maintain one's overall health and well-being.

Finally, advocacy involves supporting others who are affected by prostate cancer. This can include participating in support groups, offering emotional support and practical assistance to others who are undergoing treatment, and sharing one's personal experience to offer hope and encouragement to others.

In summary, advocacy is a critical aspect of the prostate cancer trip. By becoming informed, promoting awareness, influencing policy and practice changes, being an active participant in one's care, and supporting others, individuals can make a meaningful difference in the lives of those affected by prostate cancer.

Prostate Cancer Research and Advocacy Organizations

There are many organizations dedicated to prostate cancer research and advocacy. These organizations provide resources for patients and their families, advocate for increased funding for research, and work to raise awareness about prostate cancer and the importance of early detection.

One such organization is the Prostate Cancer Foundation (PCF). The PCF is the world's leading humanitarian association devoted to backing prostate cancer exploration. The foundation works to accelerate the development of better treatments and ultimately find a cure for prostate cancer.

The PCF also provides resources for patients and their families, including a helpline and a comprehensive online resource center. Another organization is Us TOO International, which is a nonprofit organization that provides support, education, and advocacy for men with prostate cancer and their families.

The organization offers a variety of programs and services, including a toll-free support hotline, online support groups, and educational resources.

The American Cancer Society (ACS) is another well-known organization that provides resources and support for patients with prostate cancer. The ACS offers information about the disease, treatment options, and survivorship. They also offer a variety of support programs, including a helpline and online support groups.

The Prostate Cancer Research Institute(PCRI) is a nonprofit association that's devoted to perfecting the quality of life for prostate cancer cases and their families through education and exploration. The PCRI offers a variety of resources, including educational videos, a patient conference, and a helpline staffed by medical professionals.

The Prostate Cancer Education Council (PCEC) is another organization that provides resources and education about prostate cancer. The PCEC offers free prostate cancer screenings, as well as educational programs and support groups.

Overall, these organizations play a critical role in supporting patients with prostate cancer and their families, as well as advocating for increased funding for research and raising awareness about the importance of early detection.

Staying Up-to-Date on Prostate Cancer News and Research

Staying up-to-date on prostate cancer news and research is important for both patients and caregivers. It allows them to make informed decisions about treatment options and to stay informed about advances in care.

There are several resources available for staying informed about prostate cancer news and research. One of the best sources of information is the National Cancer Institute (NCI), which is part of the National Institutes of Health (NIH).

The NCI provides information on the latest advances in prostate cancer research, as well as clinical trials that are currently recruiting patients.

Another great resource for staying informed about prostate cancer research is the Prostate Cancer Foundation (PCF). The PCF is a non-profit organization that is dedicated to funding research to find better treatments and ultimately a cure for prostate cancer.

They provide updates on the latest research findings and clinical trials, as well as information on support services for patients and families. In addition to these organizations, there are many online forums and discussion groups that allow patients and caregivers to connect with others who are going through similar experiences.

These forums can provide a valuable source of support and information, as well as a way to stay informed about the latest news and research. It's important to note that not all sources of information are reliable, and patients and caregivers should be cautious about where they get their information. It's always a good idea to check the source of the information and to talk to a healthcare professional before making any decisions about treatment options.

In summary, staying up-to-date on prostate cancer news and research is important for patients and caregivers. There are many resources available, including the NCI, PCF, and online forums, that can provide valuable information and support. However, it's important to be cautious about where information is coming from and to talk to a healthcare professional before making any decisions about treatment options.

Chapter 9

Resources for Prostate Cancer Survivors: Financial Assistance and Insurance

Prostate cancer treatment can be expensive, and the cost can sometimes be a burden on patients and their families. It is important to understand the potential costs of treatment and to explore options for financial assistance and insurance coverage.

Many health insurance plans cover the cost of prostate cancer treatment, but it is important to carefully review your plan and understand the out-of-pocket expenses that may be required. Some insurance plans may have limitations on the types of treatments that are covered or may require pre-authorization before treatment can be initiated.

Financial assistance programs are available to help patients with the cost of treatment. These programs may be offered by government agencies, nonprofit organizations, or pharmaceutical companies. Patients can also explore options for medical grants, co-pay assistance, or financial aid for prescription medications.

It is important to be aware of the potential financial impact of prostate cancer treatment and to seek out available resources for assistance. This can help alleviate the stress and burden of medical bills and allow patients to focus on their recovery and well-being.

In addition to financial assistance, patients can also take steps to minimize their out-of-pocket expenses by exploring options for generic medications, negotiating with providers for lower costs, or choosing treatment facilities that offer more affordable care.

Overall, patients and their families need to be proactive in understanding the potential costs of prostate cancer treatment and exploring options for financial assistance and insurance coverage. By taking these steps, patients can focus on their recovery and well-being without the added stress of financial burden.

Legal and Employment Issues

A prostate cancer diagnosis can have significant legal and employment implications for patients and their families. Treatment for prostate cancer may require time off work, which can result in lost wages or job loss. Additionally, treatment-related side effects, such as fatigue and difficulty concentrating, can impact job performance and limit employment opportunities.

Patients and their loved ones need to understand their legal rights and options regarding employment and finances. The following are some legal and employment issues that individuals with prostate cancer may face:

1. Disability Benefits: Patients who are unable to work due to their prostate cancer diagnosis or treatment may be eligible for disability benefits through Social Security or private disability insurance. It is important to understand the eligibility requirements and application process for these benefits.

2. Family and Medical Leave Act (FMLA): The FMLA provides eligible employees with up to 12 weeks of unpaid leave per year for medical reasons, including cancer treatment. It is important to understand the requirements for eligibility and job protection.

3. Workplace Accommodations: Employers are required to make reasonable accommodations for employees with disabilities, including those related to cancer treatment. This may include modified work schedules, flexible hours, or temporary job reassignments.

4. Discrimination: It is illegal for employers to discriminate against employees or job applicants based on their cancer diagnosis or treatment. This includes discrimination in hiring, firing, promotions, and other employment decisions.

5. Estate Planning: Individuals with prostate cancer may want to consider updating their estate plans, including wills, trusts, and power of attorney documents, to ensure their wishes are carried out in the event of their death or incapacity.

It is recommended that patients and their loved ones consult with a qualified attorney who specializes in cancer-related legal issues to understand their rights and options. Additionally, many cancer support organizations offer free legal and financial counseling services to patients and their families.

Transportation and Lodging

Transportation and lodging can be a concern for prostate cancer patients who need to travel for treatment or medical appointments. Many cancer treatment centers offer transportation services for patients who are unable to drive or need assistance getting to appointments. This can include shuttle services, volunteer drivers, and even taxis, or ride-sharing services. Patients should check with their treatment center to see what options are available.

In addition, some organizations offer lodging assistance for patients and their families who need to travel for treatment. For example, the American Cancer Society operates Hope Lodge facilities throughout the country, which provide free temporary housing for cancer patients and their caregivers. Other organizations, such as the National Patient Travel Center, assist with transportation and lodging expenses for those who meet certain eligibility criteria.

Patients and their families can also reach out to local support groups or nonprofits to see if they offer assistance with transportation or lodging. Churches, civic organizations, and even businesses in the community may also be willing to help.

For patients who can drive, it's important to make sure they are comfortable behind the wheel. Prostate cancer and its treatments can cause side effects that affect driving, such as fatigue or bladder control issues. Patients should talk to their doctor about any concerns they have and ask for recommendations on how to manage these side effects while driving.

Overall, prostate cancer patients need to plan and explore their options for transportation and lodging. By taking advantage of available resources, patients can focus on their treatment and recovery without the added stress of logistical concerns.

Chapter 10

Inspiring Survivor Stories

Prostate cancer is a challenging disease that can impact anyone, regardless of age, race, or background. However, there are countless inspiring stories of survivors who have overcome the odds and are living healthy, fulfilling lives. These stories can be a source of hope and encouragement for those who are currently battling the disease and their loved ones. Here are just a few inspiring survivor stories:

1. Arnold Palmer

Arnold Palmer, a legendary golfer, was diagnosed with prostate cancer in 1997. He underwent successful surgery and radiation treatment and went on to become a vocal advocate for prostate cancer awareness and research. He passed away in 2016 at the age of 87, but his legacy continues to inspire many.

2. Joe Torre

Joe Torre was a former Major League Baseball player and manager and was diagnosed with prostate cancer in 1999. He underwent successful surgery and has been cancer-free ever since. He has since become an advocate for prostate cancer awareness and founded the Joe Torre Safe at Home Foundation, which helps children affected by domestic violence.

3. Dan Winters

Dan Winters, a photographer, was diagnosed with prostate cancer at the age of 42. He underwent surgery and radiation treatment and has been cancer-free for over a decade. He has since become an advocate for prostate cancer awareness and founded the Winters Cancer Fund, which supports cancer research and patient care.

4. Harry Belafonte

Harry Belafonte, a singer, and actor, was diagnosed with prostate cancer in 1996. He underwent successful treatment and has been cancer-free ever since. He has since become an advocate for prostate cancer awareness and founded the Harry Belafonte 115th Street Library, which provides educational resources for underprivileged children.

5. Michael Milken

Michael Milken, a financier, and philanthropist, was diagnosed with prostate cancer in 1993. He underwent successful treatment and has been cancer-free ever since. He has since become an advocate for prostate cancer awareness and founded the Prostate Cancer Foundation, which supports prostate cancer research.

6. Samuel L. Jackson

Samuel L. Jackson, an actor, was diagnosed with prostate cancer in 2011. He underwent successful treatment and has been cancer-free ever since. He has since become an advocate for prostate cancer awareness and encourages men to get screened for the disease.

7. Colin Powell

Colin Powell, a retired four-star general and former Secretary of State, was diagnosed with prostate cancer in 2003. He underwent successful treatment and has been cancer-free ever since. He has since become an advocate for prostate cancer awareness and encourages men to get screened for the disease.

These survivors and many others have shown that prostate cancer can be overcome with early detection, proper treatment, and a positive attitude. Their stories are a testament to the power of hope and the resilience of the human spirit. By sharing their experiences, they inspire others to seek help, take action, and never give up.

Conclusion

Prostate cancer is a serious condition that can be challenging to deal with physically, emotionally, and financially. However, with advancements in medical technology and increased awareness, the survival rates for prostate cancer have improved significantly in recent years. Patients need to take an active role in their treatment and care, as well as seek support from loved ones and professional organizations.

There are many treatment options available for prostate cancer, including surgery, radiation therapy, hormone therapy, chemotherapy, and watchful waiting or active surveillance. Each treatment has its own set of benefits and potential side effects, and patients should work closely with their healthcare team to determine the best course of action for their situation.

While undergoing treatment, patients may experience a variety of side effects such as urinary incontinence, erectile dysfunction, hot flashes, and fatigue. However, there are many strategies available to help manage these side effects, including nutrition and diet, exercise and physical activity, stress management and relaxation techniques, and support groups and counseling.

It is also important for patients to stay up-to-date on the latest research and news related to prostate cancer, and to advocate for themselves and others in the prostate cancer community. There are many organizations and resources available to provide financial assistance, legal and employment guidance, and transportation and lodging support for those undergoing treatment.

Finally, it is important to remember that prostate cancer does not have to define a person's life or limit their potential. Many prostate cancer survivors have gone on to live full and inspiring lives, sharing their stories of hope and inspiration with others in the prostate cancer community. By staying informed, seeking support, and staying positive, prostate cancer patients can take an active role in their treatment and care, and continue to live fulfilling and meaningful lives.

Printed in Great Britain
by Amazon